I0536135

A Turning Point

In the depths of my frustration, a flicker of hope ignited within me. I realized that the key to my weight loss journey lay not in the hands of deceitful companies, but within my own hands and determination. I began to learn as much as I could and exploring the intricacies of weight loss.

An Epiphany

Through this journey of self discovery, I stumbled upon the realization weight loss was not a one-size fits all, Instead it demanded a deep understanding of my own body , how it works, its unique needs, and the underlying bad habits that contributing to my weight gain. I became obsessed with physical and emotional well-being, recognizing that lasting weight loss went far beyond mere numbers on a scale.

Embracing My Journey

With renewed vigor, I embarked on a journey that encompassed more than just shedding pounds. I cultivated a compassionate relationship with my body, celebrating its strength and resilience. I embraced mindful eating, savoring each bite and nurturing a deeper connection with the nourishment that fueled my being. Exercise transformed from a dreaded chore into a joyful expression of self-care, weaving into the fabric of my daily life.

Unveiling the Secret

In my mid 50s, I stand here as a living testament to the power of perseverance. Through trial and errors, I unraveled the secret to lasting weight loss, hidden within the massives different diets lies the truth. The truth lies not in restrictive diets or fleeting trends, but in the harmonious balance of nutrition, exercise, and the willingness to think differently about the food you eat. I wish to share with each and every reader who joins me on this journeyhow I won the battle.

Conclusion

As you embark on the pages that lie ahead, know that you are not alone. Together, we will navigate the winding path towards lasting weight loss, armed with knowledge, self-awareness, and the unwavering determination to win the battle. Let this book give you the encouragement, knowledge and strength to write your own story of weight loss and embrace a healthier, more fulfilled life.

I'm hopeful you will find within the pages what you need to succeed on this deeply personal journey towards lasting weight loss. I will delve into the depths of my struggles. and how I have emerged victorious, armed with knowledge, resilience, and an unyielding spirit, you can to.

As someone who has battled weight issues throughout my life, I intimately understand the challenges, the disappointments, and the relentless pursuit of a solution that truly works. It feels like I have tried every weight loss company and diet out there, hoping against hope that this time, it would be different. But each experience left me disappointed in myself and blaming myself, questioning whether I would ever find the answer.

But then, a flicker of hope ignited within me, and I realized that the power to transforming my life resided within me all along. It was not about the latest fad diet or the flashy promises of weight loss companies. No it was the relationship I had with food, I had to change my unhealthy habits. I had to discover why food was giving me life but also killing me.

Throughout my research, countless hours of self reflection, and missteps along the way, I've learnt one important lesson that you need knowledge to win this battle.

At first I struggled to understand the intricacies of metabolism, the impact of different foods had. The role of exercise, and the choices that would support my weight loss goals.

The frustrations I have endured was endless! The yo-yoing of weight loss and gain, the discouragement when the scale refused to budge, and the toll it took on my self esteem and self confidence. But with every setback, I grew stronger, more determined to find a solution that would truly endure.

So here we are, standing at the precipice of transformation. As you read through the pages of this book, I will be trying to enlighten you,and sharing the invaluable lessons I've learned. Together, we will uncover the truth of weight loss companies,and how to recognizing their short-sighted approaches and the lack of lasting results.

But fear not, for within these pages lies a beacon of hope. I will reveal to you a diet plan that actually work, a plan that respects your body's unique needs. We willlook at diet plans, recipes and how the body works.

The recipes I will list will be filled with nourishing ingredients and tantalizing flavors that will make your taste buds dance with joy hopefully hopefully.Disclaimer I'm not Gordon Ramsay.

So by the time you reach the final chapter, my hope is that you will emerge not only with a newfound knowledge and understanding of your body.Hopefully you will realize that you are not at the mercy of weight loss companies or societal expectations. No you hold the power within you to sculpt your own path to lasting weight loss.

So if you are will start on this intimate and transformative journey . the truth will support you every step of the way. Celebrate the victories, navigate the challenges, and emerge as resilient warriors, armed with the knowledge and confidence to create lasting change in our lives.

Chapter 1

The Truth About Diet Companies and Their Rip-Offs

Let's get real for a moment. We've all heard the enticing promises of the diet industry, the quick fixes, the perfect bodies and how your dreams can come true for a price of course. But as many of us have come to discover, the reality is far from what they promised. It's a world filled with disappointment, frustration, and financial loss. It seems like these companies are more interested in filling their pockets than actually helping us achieve our goals, well why kill the Golden Goose.

In this chapter of the book, i will try and shine a light on the shady side of these weight loss companies. A wake-up call to be more sceptical and discerning when it comes to choosing a diet plan or product. I will explore the studies also the truth behind these companies, their efficacy, their limitations, and the impact they have on our lives, mental health and self-esteem.

If you've ever tried to lose weight or become a little bit more healthy, chances are you've encountered a quite a few of these diet companies.

They are everywhere and not in a good way, from flashy TV ads to magazine spreads and even online ads. These companies promise you the moon, but sadly, there many goal is just out to rip you off.

I'll speak honestly these weight loss companies are a massive business, raking in billions of dollars each year. With that kind of money at stake, it's no wonder that some companies put their profits over your well being. They'll use every trick in the book to your money , but the truth is, most of their diets aren't sustainable, healthy, or effective in the long run.

Some of the biggest tactics they use to pull the wool over your eyes is by selling diets based on questionable science and bogus claims. But these claims often lack scientific evidence, and many people end up losing weight only to see it come right back because these products they sell are not designed to work in a long term, they designed for repeat business.

And let's not forget about those pricey supplements, shakes, and other products they push. While some of them may offer a few benefits.

They aren't necessary for weight loss and are overpriced for what they are. On top of that, some of these products hide sketchy ingredients or haven't undergone proper safety testing at all.

But here's the real kicker these con artists often sell you one-size-fits-all weight loss programs that simply don't cater to your unique needs. Unfortunately, these companies want you to believe that the only way to keep losing weight is to keep paying even if you are experiencing disappointing results.

It is so crucial to recognize that the weight loss industry is more focused on making money.if there was no money in the industry they would not exist just take a moment to think about this. They'll employ clever marketing tactics to draw you in, selling you fad diets, overpriced supplements, and weight loss programs that simply don't work.

So with this knowledge, you can make an conscious decisions about your goals . You don't have to fall for their tricks you can stand strong, take back control and treat these people with the contempt they deserve.

Remember, you're in charge of your own health journey, no one else. So approach weight loss with a critical eye, focusing not just on shedding pounds but on overall health and wellness. By doing this, you will rise above the misleading tactics of these weight loss companies and find our path to enlightenment and happiness.

So trust in yourself to know what is best for you and armed with the knowledge that we are just looked at as cash cows by the weight loss industry , trust your instincts, and let's embark on this journey.

Chapter 2

All Calories Are Not Equal

I want to talk about calories and weight loss.This is a very important topic that we have to cover because not all calories are equal. While calories measure the energy in our food, where those calories come from can make a significant difference in our weight loss journey.

You you will be aware of the concept of calorie counting, keep track of the calories you take in compared to the calories you burn off. While it can be a helpful , some experts argue that calorie counting alone is not the most effective method for weight loss. It overlooks importants of the quality of the calories consumed and the role of hormones and metabolism.Because 200 calories of chocolate is not the same as 200 calories of carrots.

So here come a boring bit this is where the research comes in. Numerous studies have shed light on the impact of macronutrient composition and the quality of calories on weight loss and overall health. Let's explore a few of these studies.

A review published in the Annual Review of Nutrition in 2015 analyzed 29 randomized controlled trials. The review found that diets higher in protein and lower in carbohydrates or fat were more effective for weight loss and improving metabolic health markers than diets low in protein. The study highlighted the importance of considering macronutrient balance in achieving weight loss goals.

In a study published in the Journal of the American Medical Association in 2012, overweight and obese individuals were divided into two groups. One group followed a low-carbohydrate diet (with more calories from fat and protein),

while the other followed a low-fat diet (with fewer calories from fat). Interestingly, despite consuming the same number of calories, the low carbohydrate group experienced greater weight loss and improvements in health markers.

Another study published in the International Journal of Obesity in 2014 compared the effects of a high-protein, low-carbohydrate diet to a high carbohydrate, low-protein diet in overweight and obese individuals.

Both groups consumed the same number of calories, yet the high protein group lost more body fat and preserved more lean muscle mass. These findings suggest that the quality of calories, specifically the macronutrient composition, plays a crucial role in weight loss and body composition changes.

These studies highlight the significance of considering the quality of the calories we consume, rather than solely focusing on the quantity. While calorie counting can be a useful tool for weight management, it is essential to understand that not all calories are equal when it comes to their impact on our health and weight.

However, it's crucial to acknowledge the potential downsides of calorie counting as well. Here are a few points to consider.

Counting calories needs careful tracking and measuring of everything you eat and drink, which can be a complete pain. This aspect may not be sustainable for everyone,in fact it can leading to frustration and a discontinuation of the diet that you are following.

Unhealthy focus on numbers and not what you are putting in your mouth can sometimes can manifests itself in to an unhealthy preoccupation with the numbers on the scale or in food labels. This can lead to bad eating habits and an unhealthy relationship with food.

While calorie counting can help manage weight, it dose not address underlying issues that contribute to overeating or an unhealthy relationship with food.

Calorie counting is often used as a short-term weight loss strategy. However, maintaining long term weight loss is very difficult with this method. The potential to slip back into old eating habits is very high,That is why I don't particularly recommend using calorie counting for weight loss I believe there are better alternatives for your weight loss journey and strategies that can be used over the long-term to better effect.

Here are some examples to illustrate how not all calories are equal

Protein vs. Processed Foods: Let's compare 100 calories of grilled chicken breast to 100 calories of potato chips or crisp if your in the uk. While both may have the same number of calories, the grilled chicken breast is a lean source of protein that provides essential amino acids and contributes to satiety. On the other hand, potato chips are highly processed, lacking essential nutrients and fiber. They are high in unhealthy fats and often lead to overeating due to their addictive nature.

Whole Grains vs. Refined Grains: Consider 100 calories of whole wheat bread versus 100 calories of white bread. Whole wheat bread is a complex carbohydrate that provides fiber, vitamins, and minerals. It helps regulate blood sugar levels and keeps you feeling fuller for longer.

In contrast, white bread is made from refined grains, stripped of their fiber and nutrients. It can cause blood sugar spikes and lead to cravings and overeating.This will also lead to a spike in insulin and when insulin is prevalent in the body you cannot burn fat instantly is a fat storing hormone but we'll cover this later.

Fruits vs. Sugary Drinks: Take 100 calories of fresh strawberries versus 100 calories of a sugary soda.This really is a no brainer strawberries are packed with vitamins, minerals.In contrast, the sugary soda is devoid of nutritional value, providing empty calories that can spike blood sugar levels and will help you gain weight.

These examples demonstrate that even if two food items have the same number of calories, their nutritional composition will impact on our bodies Indifferent ways. It's important to eat whole foods over processed and sugary options for long-term health and sustainable weight loss.

Focusing on the quality of calories, you can Feed your body with good calories instead of bad calories. Your body needs good nutrients while on your weightloss journey, if you think of your body as a car,if you put bad petrol into it the car won't perform properly and your body is the same put good nutrients in and your body will thank you.

Let's move beyond the idea that all calories are equal. By making mindful choices and embracing a balanced approach to nutrition, you can achieve sustainable weight loss and enjoy the numerous health benefits that come with it.

Chapter 3

Unraveling the Mysteries of Carbohydrates and Their Impact on Weight Loss

Let's dive into the fascinating world of carbohydrates. They're a fundamental part of our diet, by understanding how they work in our bodies can greatly impact our weight loss journey. In this chapter, we will try to explore where carbohydrates are found in food, how the body stores them, and the some of the benefits of low-carbohydrate diets. So I want to try to explain why I think that a low-carb diet is basically the way to go to lose weight constantly and for the long term. So make yourself comfortable let's cover carbohydrates .

Carbohydrates are found in lots of foods such as grains, fruits, vegetables, legumes, and dairy products. They serve as the body's primary source of energy. When eaten , our body breaks them down into glucose, which fuels our cells and provides energy for our daily activities.

Once carbohydrates are broken down into glucose, our body uses what it needs for immediate energy and stores the excess for later use as fat. The primary storage form of carbohydrates is glycogen. Glycogen is stored in the liver and muscles, where it acts as a readily available energy source when needed.

But we have to understand how carbohydrates are stored as fat, As I said earlier we must explore the role of insulin, a hormone secreted by the pancreas. When we eat carbohydrates, our blood glucose levels rise. In response, the pancreas releases insulin, which takes glucose from the bloodstream into our cells.

Once inside the cells, glucose can be used for immediate energy production. However, if there is an excess amount of glucose, it undergoes a process called lipogenesis. During lipogenesis, glucose is converted into fatty acids and then stored as triglycerides, the primary form of fat storage in our bodies.So the science says if you eat excess carbohydrates they will store as fat,this is a problem when trying to lose weight. Calorie control diets don't take this into account.

Medical studies provide valuable insights into the impact of carbohydrates on weight loss.So you're thinking I haven't bought this book to read medical studies, but they are important to understand what's happening with your body.Here are a few studies that shed light on this topic and they won't take too long to read through.

A study published in the New England Journal of Medicine compared low carbohydrate and low fat diets .So how many times have you been told to use a low-fat diet by a so-called dietitian or a doctor.The study found that participants on the low carbohydrate diet had greater weight loss and improvements in heart disease risk factors compared to those on the low-fat diet.This is because some studies show that some fats are good for the heart.

Another study published in the Annals of Internal Medicine examined the effects of a low carbohydrate ketogenic diet .Ok so we've all heard of the keto diet. The study reported that participants following the keto diet lost more weight and experienced greater improvements in insulin sensitivity compared to those on a low-fat diet.So what we've been told for years is completely wrong.

Low carb diets have gained popularity for their potential benefits in weight loss. Here's how they can contribute to your weight loss journey.

So when we eat fewer carb, your body turns to stored fat as an alternative fuel source. This can promote increased fat burning and will Improved Blood Sugar Control.

Low carb diets can help stabilize blood sugars, reducing insulin spikes and promoting better blood sugar control because carbohydrates increase sugars In the blood .So eating a low carb diet means lower blood sugar, this can be particularly beneficial for individuals with insulin resistance or diabetes.

Foods rich in carb can sometimes leave us feeling hungry soon after eating due to rapid blood sugar spikes and subsequent crashes. Low carb diets, often rich in protein and healthy fats, can promote feeling of Being full for longer Which can reducing the urge to overeat.

Now just a little bit about high triglyceride levels In your body.It is not a good idea to have high levels of triglyceride in the blood as it is associated with an increased risk of heart disease.

Research suggests that low carb diets can lower triglyceride levels, thereby promoting heart health.

Now with the knowledge that carbohydrates and their impact on weight loss can be a game changer and it's in your hands . By eating carb mindfully and considering the benefits of low carb diets, you can win the battle in your weight loss journey. Remember, everyone's body is different but the science is the science, so finding the approach that works best for you is key.

So embrace the power of low carb diets, make informed choices, and explore its benefits . With knowledge as our ally, you now know why you have gained weight.Changing the way you think about carbs will unlock the secrets to successful weight loss and pave the way to. Victory!

Chapter 4

The Gut Microbiome

The gut microbiome plays an important role in human health by performing various functions such as breaking down dietary fibers, producing vitamins and other important molecules, and interacting with the immune system. A healthy and diverse gut microbiome is crucial for maintaining good overall health, including digestive health, immune function, and mental health. On the other hand, an imbalance in the gut microbiome, known as dysbiosis, has been linked to a range of health issues, including inflammatory bowel disease, allergies, and even some neurological disorders.

Alcohol consumption can have a negative impact on the gut microbiome by disrupting the balance of beneficial bacteria and potentially promoting the growth of harmful bacteria. I know most of us like a little drink and now and then, but excessive drinking can lead to inflammation and damage to the gut lining, and may increase the risk of certain gut-related health issues, such as leaky gut syndrome and irritable bowel syndrome.

Long term excessive alcohol consumption may also increase the risk of developing certain types of cancers, such as colon cancer.

Consuming a diet high in processed foods can also have negative effects on the gut microbiome. Processed foods are often high in added sugars, artificial ingredients, and preservatives, and low in fiber, which can disrupt the balance of beneficial bacteria in the gut. Additionally,

a diet high in processed foods has been linked to an increased risk of developing chronic diseases such as obesity, type 2 diabetes and heart disease. Processed food can also increase inflammation in the gut and can lead to gut-related issues such as leaky gut syndrome and irritable bowel syndrome.

Foods that are good for the gut include those that are high in fiber, prebiotics, and probiotics. Fiber is important for maintaining a healthy gut because it helps to keep the digestive system regular and promotes the growth of beneficial bacteria. High-fiber foods include fruits, vegetables, whole grains, and legumes.

Prebiotics are non-digestible carbohydrates that promote the growth of beneficial bacteria in the gut. Some examples of foods high in prebiotics include onions, garlic, leeks, asparagus, bananas, oats, and apples.

Probiotics are beneficial bacteria that can be found in fermented foods such as yogurt, kefir, sauerkraut, kimchi, kombucha, and miso.

High-fiber fruits and vegetables: apples, berries, avocados, artichokes, broccoli, Brussels sprouts, leafy greens.

Whole grains: oats, quinoa, brown rice, barley.

Legumes: lentils, chickpeas, beans, peas.

Fermented foods: yogurt, kefir, sauerkraut, kimchi, kombucha, miso.

Nuts and seeds: almonds, flaxseed, chia seeds, pumpkin seeds.

Bone broth.

Extra virgin olive oil.

Fatty fish: salmon, mackerel, sardine.

Foods high in prebiotics: onions, garlic, leeks, asparagus, bananas, oats, apples.

A healthy gut microbiome has been linked to a variety of health benefits, including.

Improved digestion: A diverse and balanced gut microbiome can aid in the breakdown and absorption of nutrients from food, which can lead to better digestion and regular bowel movements.

A stronger immune system: A healthy gut microbiome can help to support the immune system by producing antibodies and other molecules that can help to protect against harmful pathogens.

Reduced inflammation: A healthy gut microbiome can help to reduce inflammation throughout the body, which may reduce the risk of certain chronic diseases such as heart disease, type 2 diabetes and certain types of cancer.

A healthy gut microbiome has been linked to a better mood and reduced risk of anxiety and depression.

Weight management: A healthy gut microbiome has been linked to weight management by helping to regulate appetite and metabolism.

Better skin health: A healthy gut microbiome has been linked to improved skin health, it can help to reduce inflammation and promote a clear complexion.

It's important to note that a healthy gut is one aspect of overall health and well-being, and it's important to maintain a healthy lifestyle by eating a balanced diet, exercising regularly, and reducing stress.

Remember, a healthy gut diet is a well-rounded and balanced diet with a variety of nutrient-dense foods. It's important to eat a variety of all foods, and not just focus on one type of food.

Tim Spector is a professor at King's College London. He is a professor of genetic epidemiology and the director of the TwinsUK Registry, a research project that studies the health and genetics of twins in the UK. Spector has also held academic positions at several other universities, including St. Thomas' Hospital, the University of Surrey, and the University of Western Australia.

Professor Tim Spector is also a British author who is known for his research on the human microbiome and its impact on health. He is the author of several books, including "The Diet Myth: The Real Science Behind What We Eat," in which he argues that the diversity of microbes in the gut is crucial for overall health and that a varied diet is necessary for maintaining that diversity.

Professor Spector's research has focused on the role of the microbiome in various health conditions, including obesity, mental health, and autoimmune diseases. He has also been an advocate for the use of personalized diets based on an individual's unique microbiome composition.

Structure, function and diversity of the healthy human microbiome" by Huttenhower et al., published in Nature in 2012.

Diet-induced extinctions in the gut microbiota compound over generations" by Sonnenburg et al., published in Nature in 2016.

Antibiotics, gut microbiota, and obesity" by Cho et al., published in The Lancet in 2012.

The gut microbiome and its role in obesity" by
Turnbaugh et al., published in Cell in 2006.

The gut-brain axis: interactions between enteric
microbiota, central and enteric nervous
systems" by Cryan and Dinan, published in
Annals of the New York Academy of Sciences in
2012.

Chapter 5

Unraveling the Role of Hormones in Weight Gain and the Benefits of Low-Carbohydrate Diets

Today, we're delving into the fascinating world of hormones and their influence on weight gain. You see, for the longest time, I struggled with weight gain and felt helpless and depressed about not realizing the significant role hormones play in this journey. But fear not, for you about to start on a journey of discovery . In this chapter, we'll explore the intricate connection between hormones and weight gain, focusing on key hormones like ghrelin, insulin, cortisol, adrenaline, and leptin. We'll also unravel the benefits of low-carbohydrate diets for weight loss. So, let's dive in with open a mind.

Let's start by getting acquainted with some of the major hormones that can impact weight gain.

Ghrelin: This hormone, produced by specialized cells in the stomach, plays a crucial role in regulating hunger and food intake.

Ghrelin levels increase before meals and decrease after eating. It stimulates appetite and food intake, promoting the storage of fat and potentially leading to weight gain. Research has also shown that ghrelin can impact glucose metabolism and insulin response, further influencing weight management.

Ghrelin also plays a role in regulating body weight. Ghrelin promotes the storage of fat and decreases energy expenditure, which can lead to weight gain if ghrelin levels are too high or if the body is unable to respond properly to ghrelin. Ghrelin also has a role in the regulation of glucose metabolism and the insulin response, which can affect the body's ability to regulate blood sugar levels.

In addition to its role in hunger and metabolism, ghrelin also has been found to have effects on other physiological functions such as cardiovascular function, immunity, and stress response. Ghrelin has also been found to play a role in certain diseases such as obesity, diabetes, and cancer.

Ghrelin levels are decreased in some disorders such as anorexia nervosa, and increased in others such as Prader-Willi syndrome. Ghrelin levels also decrease with aging.

Prader-Willi syndrome (PWS) is a genetic disorder that can lead to insatiable hunger and an intense craving for food. This can often lead to the development of an eating disorder, such as hyperphagia and obesity.

Hyperphagia is the term used to describe the constant feeling of hunger and the desire to eat, even after having just eaten. People with PWS have difficulty feeling full, and their hunger is not regulated by the normal mechanisms in the brain that control appetite. This can lead to binge eating, which can be dangerous as it can lead to obesity and related health problems such as heart disease, diabetes, and respiratory problems.

It's important to note that each individual with PWS may have different symptoms and needs, so treatment plans should be tailored to the individual. In addition to dietary and lifestyle interventions, individuals with PWS may also benefit from therapy and support to address the emotional and behavioral issues associated with the disorder.

Research is ongoing to better understand the role of ghrelin in the body and the potential for using ghrelin or drugs that target ghrelin as a treatment for conditions such as obesity, eating disorders, and diabetes.

Insulin: The hormone insulin is a key player in the body's metabolism and energy balance. It helps transport glucose from the bloodstream into cells for energy or storage. Excess glucose that cannot be immediately used is converted into fat and stored in adipose tissue. High insulin levels, often resulting from a diet high in carbohydrates and added sugars, can contribute to weight gain and obesity over time. Insulin resistance, a condition where cells do not respond properly to insulin, can further complicate weight management and increase the risk of type 2 diabetes.

Insulin resistance is a condition in which the body's cells do not respond properly to insulin, which leads to higher insulin levels, increased fat storage, and difficulty in losing weight. It is also a risk factor for type 2 diabetes.

Type 2 diabetes is a chronic condition in which the body's cells do not respond properly to insulin, resulting in high blood sugar levels.

It is the most common form of diabetes and is often associated with obesity, physical inactivity, and a diet high in carbohydrates and added sugars.

In type 2 diabetes, the pancreas still produces insulin, but the body's cells do not respond to it properly, a condition known as insulin resistance. This leads to higher insulin levels in the blood, which can cause the pancreas to produce even more insulin. Over time, the pancreas may not be able to keep up with the body's demands for insulin, leading to decreased insulin production and even higher blood sugar levels.

Type 2 diabetes is a progressive disease, and it can take years for it to develop. Initially, the body can compensate for the insulin resistance by producing more insulin, but eventually, the pancreas can't keep up, and blood sugar levels rise.

The main goal of treatment for type 2 diabetes is to lower blood sugar levels and prevent the development of diabetes-related complications, such as heart disease, kidney disease, nerve damage, and eye problems.

Treatment options include lifestyle changes, such as a healthy diet and regular physical activity, as well as medications to lower blood sugar levels, such as metformin and sulfonylureas. In some cases, insulin therapy may also be required.

It's essential to address a common misconception related to the term "pre-diabetic." When a doctor tells you that you're pre-diabetic, it doesn't necessarily mean you're overweight or fat. Pre-diabetes refers to a condition where blood sugar levels are higher than normal but not yet in the diabetic range. It serves as a warning sign, highlighting the need for proactive measures to prevent or delay the onset of type 2 diabetes.

It's crucial to understand that pre-diabetes can affect individuals of various body sizes and shapes. While excess weight is a known risk factor for type 2 diabetes, genetics, lifestyle, and other factors also play a significant role. The medical community recognizes the importance of adopting a holistic approach to diabetes prevention and management, focusing on overall health rather than solely weight.

So, if you've been labeled as pre-diabetic, remember that it's not an indication of your worth or solely tied to your body size. It's an opportunity to prioritize your health and make positive changes in your lifestyle, regardless of your weight. Embrace your body, focus on nourishing it with balanced nutrition, staying active, and seeking support from healthcare professionals who take a comprehensive and individualized approach to your well-being.

Improved Hormonal Balance: Low-carbohydrate diets may positively influence hormones involved in weight regulation. They can help reduce ghrelin levels, the hunger hormone, leading to decreased appetite and improved portion control. Additionally, these diets can help regulate insulin levels, reducing the risk of insulin resistance and promoting better blood sugar control.

Growth hormone (GH) is a hormone that is produced and secreted by the pituitary gland in the brain. It plays a key role in growth, metabolism, and body composition. GH stimulates the growth of bone, muscle, and other tissues, and it also helps to regulate metabolism by promoting the breakdown of fat cells and the release of glucose into the bloodstream. In addition,

GH is involved in regulating the immune system and maintaining bone density. GH levels are highest during childhood and adolescence and gradually decrease as we age.

Abnormal GH levels can lead to various health problems, including growth disorders and metabolic disorders such as diabetes.

Cortisol is a hormone that is produced by the adrenal glands in response to stress. It is often referred to as the "stress hormone" because it plays a key role in the body's stress response.

Cortisol has many important functions in the body, including the regulation of blood sugar levels, blood pressure, and immune function. It also plays a role in the body's metabolism of carbohydrates, fats, and proteins.

Leptin is a hormone produced by adipose (fat) tissue in the body that plays a key role in regulating body weight and energy balance. It acts on the hypothalamus, a region of the brain that controls appetite and metabolism, to reduce food intake and increase energy expenditure.

Leptin levels increase as body fat increases, and high levels of leptin signal the brain to decrease appetite and increase energy expenditure.

Conversely, low levels of leptin signal the brain to increase appetite and decrease energy expenditure.

Leptin also has other functions in the body, such as regulating reproductive function and immune function. Leptin resistance, a condition where the body becomes less responsive to leptin, can contribute to obesity and other health problems.

Get enough sleep: Sleep deprivation can disrupt the production and regulation of leptin, leading to decreased levels.

Eat a balanced diet: Consuming a diet that is high in protein and fiber, and low in processed and high-sugar foods may help to regulate leptin levels and improve sensitivity.

Exercise: Regular physical activity can improve leptin sensitivity and increase leptin levels in the body.

Reduce stress: Stress can disrupt leptin regulation and lead to decreased levels. Practicing stress reduction techniques such as meditation or yoga may help to improve leptin levels.

So understanding the role of hormones in weight gain and exploring the benefits of low-carbohydrate diets can empower us on our weight loss journey. By acknowledging the influence of hormones like ghrelin, insulin, cortisol, adrenaline, and leptin, we can make informed choices to support our weight management efforts. Incorporating a low-carbohydrate diet, rich in nutrient-dense foods, can help regulate hormones.

Remember, you are so much more than a label or a number. Your health journey is unique, and by understanding the role of hormones and making informed choices, you can navigate towards a healthier and happier life. Keep striving for balance and self-care, and celebrate the diversity that makes each body remarkable in its own way.

Chapter 6

Sleep and Exercise

So in this chapter i'm going to talk a little bit about sleep and exercise, personally I only need about seven hours sleep a night, and as for exercise I generally don't like vigorous exercise but I will take a walk which is exercise, but at a moderate pace .Studies have shown that people who get enough sleep tend to have a healthier body weight than those who don't. Adequate sleep helps to regulate the hormones that control appetite, including ghrelin and leptin. If you don't get enough sleep your body produces more ghrelin (a hormone that makes you feel hungry) and less leptin (a hormone that makes you feel full). Additionally, lack of sleep can cause an increase in cortisol levels, which can lead to fat accumulation in the abdominal area.

A study published in the Journal of Clinical Sleep Medicine in 2019, which looked at data from over 2,000 adults over a period of 5 years, found that individuals who slept for less than 7 hours per night had a higher risk of becoming obese.

One study that found a link between sleep and weight loss was conducted by the University of Colorado and published in the journal "Sleep" in 2008. The study followed 68 adults who were overweight or obese and found that those who slept for 5 hours or less per night had a significantly higher body mass index (BMI) compared to those who slept for 7 hours or more. Additionally, the study found that participants who slept for 5 hours or less per night had higher levels of ghrelin and lower levels of leptin, which can lead to increased appetite and weight gain.

Another study published in the Journal of Sleep Research in 2017, found that adults who received cognitive behavioral therapy for insomnia (CBT-I) lost more weight than those who received standard weight loss therapy alone. CBT-I is a form of therapy that focuses on changing the thoughts and behaviors that can lead to insomnia, including poor sleep habits and negative beliefs about sleep. The study suggests that treating insomnia may help to improve weight loss outcomes by improving the regulation of appetite-related hormones and reducing the risk of overeating.

Overall, the studies suggest that adequate sleep is crucial for weight management and that people who have difficulty sleeping should consider seeking treatment for insomnia.

Improving sleep quality and duration can help regulate hormones that control appetite, reduce the risk of overeating, and promote healthy food choices.

Low intensity exercise is a form of physical activity that involves moderate levels of effort and can be sustained for longer periods of time. This type of exercise typically involves movements that are less vigorous and don't require as much energy as high intensity exercise.

Low intensity exercise can offer numerous benefits for people who are overweight. Here are some of the benefits.

Improved cardiovascular health: Low intensity exercise such as walking or cycling at a steady pace can help improve your cardiovascular health by strengthening your heart and improving circulation. This can reduce your risk of heart disease and stroke.

Increased mobility: Being overweight can often make movement more difficult, but regular low intensity exercise can help improve mobility and flexibility, making it easier to perform everyday tasks.

Weight loss: While low intensity exercise may not burn as many calories as high intensity exercise, it can still contribute to weight loss when combined with a healthy diet.

Reduced stress: Exercise has been shown to reduce stress and anxiety levels, which can be particularly beneficial for people who are overweight and may experience social stigma and discrimination.

Improved mood: Low intensity exercise can release endorphins, which can help improve mood and reduce feelings of depression.

Lowered risk of injury: Low intensity exercise is less likely to cause injury compared to high intensity exercise, making it a safer option for people who are overweight and may be more prone to injury.

Better sleep: Regular exercise can improve the quality of your sleep, leading to better overall health and well-being.

Examples of low intensity exercise include

Walking at a comfortable pace.

Light resistance training using weights or resistance bands.

Cycling on a stationary bike at a moderate resistance level.

Swimming or water aerobics Yoga or stretching.

Gardening or yard work.

Low intensity exercise can still provide significant health benefits, such as improving cardiovascular health, increasing mobility, reducing stress, and promoting weight loss when combined with a healthy diet. It is a good option for people who are just starting an exercise program or for those who may have physical limitations that prevent them from engaging in high intensity exercise.

Low-intensity exercise is often recommended for overweight or obese individuals because it can provide many health benefits without placing excessive stress on the joints and muscles, which can be particularly important for those who are carrying extra weight.

Studies have shown that overweight or obese individuals are more likely to stick to a low-intensity exercise program compared to high-intensity exercise. This is because low-intensity exercise is generally more enjoyable, less intimidating, and easier to perform, making it more sustainable in the long run.

Low-intensity exercise can improve insulin sensitivity, which can help to prevent or manage type 2 diabetes.

Several studies have shown that low-intensity exercise can be effective for weight loss in overweight or obese individuals. For example, a study published in the American Journal of Clinical Nutrition found that overweight individuals who walked for 60 minutes per day, five days per week, lost significant amounts of body fat over a 12-week period. Another study published in the Journal of Obesity found that overweight individuals who engaged in low-intensity cycling for 30 minutes, three times per week, experienced significant reductions in body weight and body fat over an eight week period.

A study published in the Journal of Sports Medicine and Physical Fitness found that overweight individuals who engaged in low-intensity exercise, such as walking or cycling, for 30-60 minutes, three to five times per week, experienced significant reductions in body weight, body mass index (BMI), and body fat over a 12-week period.

A study published in the Journal of Applied Physiology found that overweight individuals who engaged in low-intensity exercise, such as walking or cycling, for 45-60 minutes, three to five times per week, experienced significant reductions in visceral fat (fat around the organs) over a 12-week period.

Overall, these studies suggest that low-intensity exercise can be an effective way for overweight or obese individuals to achieve weight loss and improve their overall health. It is important to consult with a doctor or a professional before starting any exercise program, especially if you have any pre-existing medical conditions.

Chapter 7

Autophagy: Embracing Cellular Balance and Uncovering its Secrets

Now I want to discuss the topic of autophagy, which plays a critical role in maintaining cellular balance. Think of it as the body's recycling system that helps remove and recycle damaged or unnecessary components, keeping our cells healthy and functioning optimally. I think that incredible.

I had a moment of realization myself when I discovered how hormones can have a significant impact on weight gain and overall health. It's surprising how much our bodies are influenced by these chemical messengers.

Many of us have heard of the term "pre diabetic" It's often thrown around, but it's important to remember that being labeled as pre-diabetic doesn't mean you're automatically fat.In some cases pre-diabetes refers to higher than normal blood sugar levels, serving as a warning sign that lifestyle changes are needed to prevent or delay the onset of type 2 diabetes.

It's not about the number on the scale but rather about taking proactive measures to maintain our health.

Now sometimes medical professionals can use this term. At the start of my journey of weight loss I had an appointment with my doctor who will remain nameless. I was sitting in the doctors office he looked me straight in the eye and said your morbidly obese and pre-diabetic, I said really can you tell that just by looking at me , he said yes you're overweight and I replied no I mean about being pre-diabetic and he said well your overweight, I said yes but don't you think that you should do some tests on my blood before come to the conclusion that I'm pre-diabetic, so he huffed and puffed look to his computer right scribbled some notes down then said okay you can have them blood tests I said thank you.

I made a Appointment see the nurse to take some blood and two days later I had the blood test. The nurse said to me it would be about a week before the test results were in.
Well the results come back about one week later and to everybody surprise my blood sugars were normal I was completely in a normal range but if I hadn't asked for a blood test I could have been put on all sorts of medication I didn't need all.

So what is insulin and how does it affect us and why is it so important to understand its job in our body.So I'll try to explain the best I can.
When we eat, especially meals high in carbohydrates, our blood glucose levels increase. To manage this, our pancreas releases insulin, which helps transport glucose into our cells to be used for energy. But when there's an excess of glucose that our cells can't absorb, insulin promotes the storage of that excess glucose as fat in adipose tissue. That's why high insulin levels, often caused by a diet high in carbs and added sugars, can contribute to weight gain and obesity over time.

Insulin resistance is a condition where our body's cells don't respond properly to insulin, leading to higher insulin levels and difficulty in losing weight. It's also a risk factor for type 2 diabetes.

But guess what? you can take charge of your health through lifestyle changes, regardless of our body size. Making healthy food choices, staying active, and managing stress are all factors that can help improve insulin sensitivity and overall well-being.

Now, let's explore the fascinating process of autophagy. Our body has this incredible ability to activate autophagy when it's in need. It kicks in during periods of nutrient deprivation or cellular stress, helping our cells break down and recycle components for energy and cellular maintenance. Hormones like glucagon and growth hormone can trigger autophagy, especially during fasting or exercise when our body needs to tap into its own resources.

What's intriguing is that researchers are actively studying how we can harness the power of autophagy for our health. They're investigating various ways to modulate autophagy as a potential therapeutic strategy for diseases like neurodegenerative disorders, cancer, and metabolic conditions. It's truly an exciting field with promising possibilities!

And here's a little secret: fasting can be a powerful trigger for autophagy. When we fast, our body goes into a state of nutrient deprivation, lowering insulin levels and increasing hormones like glucagon.

This hormonal shift activates autophagy to break down and recycle cellular components for energy. Fascinating, isn't it?

Studies have shown that fasting can increase Autophagy in various tissues, such as the liver, muscle, and brain (Mizushima et al., 2004; Alirezaei et al., 2010; Cheng et al., 2014). For example, a study published in the journal Cell Metabolism found that intermittent fasting in mice led to increased Autophagy in the liver and improved glucose and lipid metabolism (Liu et al., 2016).

Remember, though, autophagy isn't solely triggered by fasting. Exercise is another fantastic way to stimulate autophagy in various tissues, such as our muscles and liver. Regular physical activity keeps our cells active and promotes a healthy balance within our body.

Autophagy, as we discussed earlier, is the body's way of recycling and renewing cellular components. It helps remove damaged or unnecessary components, maintaining cellular balance and function. But what does autophagy have to do with aging, you might wonder? As we

age our cells accumulate more damaged components and face greater stress from environmental factors. This can impair their function and lead to the development of age-related diseases. Here's where autophagy comes into play.

It acts as a cellular housekeeper, removing these damaged components and promoting cellular health and longevity.

Research has shown that autophagy declines as we age, which may contribute to the development of various age-related conditions. By enhancing autophagy, we may be able to slow down the aging process and potentially prevent age-related diseases.

One fascinating aspect of autophagy and aging is its impact on longevity. Studies conducted on various organisms, from yeast to worms to mice, have revealed that promoting autophagy can extend lifespan.

For example, when researchers activated autophagy genes in worms, the worms lived longer and exhibited improved health.

Similarly, calorie restriction, which is known to enhance autophagy, has been shown to increase lifespan in several species. Calorie restriction mimetics, such as the drug rapamycin, which stimulates autophagy, have also shown promising results in extending lifespan in animal studies.

But what about humans? While direct evidence linking autophagy to human lifespan is still limited, there's growing interest in understanding its role in aging and age-related diseases. Research suggests that enhancing autophagy may have anti-aging effects and protect against age-related conditions such as neurodegenerative diseases, cancer, and metabolic disorders.

Furthermore, autophagy has been found to play a role in the clearance of protein aggregates, a hallmark of many neurodegenerative diseases like Alzheimer's and Parkinson's. By eliminating these toxic aggregates, autophagy helps to maintain brain health and potentially delay the onset or progression of these diseases.

So, how can we enhance autophagy and potentially slow down the aging process? Well, it turns out that certain lifestyle factors can play a significant role.

Regular exercise has been shown to stimulate autophagy in various tissues. Engaging in physical activity not only keeps our bodies fit and healthy but also promotes cellular renewal through autophagy.

Isn't it wonderful how something as simple as exercise can have such profound effects on our cellular health and longevity?

Another strategy is maintaining a balanced and nutritious diet. Caloric restriction, which involves reducing calorie intake without malnutrition, has been linked to enhanced autophagy and longevity in various organisms. While more research is needed, adopting a mindful approach to eating, focusing on whole, nutrient-dense foods, and avoiding excessive calorie intake may support autophagy and promote healthy aging.

Now, it's important to note that autophagy is a complex process influenced by multiple factors, including genetics, lifestyle, and environmental cues. Researchers are still unraveling the intricacies of autophagy and its connection to aging.

I realize that Autophagy can be triggered by various stimuli, including nutrient deprivation, cellular stress, hormones, and exercise. One of the most well-known triggers of Autophagy is fasting, which has been shown to increase Autophagy in multiple tissues and may have potential benefits for a range of diseases and conditions.

I think Autophagy is an incredibly fascinating process because of its importance in maintaining cellular homeostasis and preventing the development of various diseases and conditions. It has been linked to a wide range of health benefits, including improved metabolism, decreased inflammation, and increased lifespan.

So, here's to embracing the wonders of autophagy and nurturing our bodies with the love and care they deserve. Let's embark on a journey of healthy aging, where each day brings us closer to uncovering the fountain of youth that lies within us.

Chapter 8

Unlocking the Benefits of Fasting Nourishing Body and Mind

Fasting, the intentional act of abstaining from food for a specific period, has been practiced for centuries for religious, cultural, and health purposes. In recent years, it has gained significant attention for its potential benefits beyond simple calorie restriction. So, let's dive into the incredible benefits that fasting can offer to nourish our bodies and minds.

So weight Loss and Metabolic Health: One of the most well known benefits of fasting is its ability to promote weight loss. When we fast, our bodies tap into stored fat for energy, leading to fat burning and ultimately shedding unwanted pounds. Additionally, fasting has been shown to improve insulin sensitivity and regulate blood sugar levels, which can be beneficial for managing conditions like type 2 diabetes.

Several studies have demonstrated the effectiveness of fasting for weight loss. For instance, a study published in JAMA Internal Medicine found that intermittent fasting resulted in significant weight loss.

Enhanced Brain Function: Fasting has also shown promise in boosting cognitive function and brain health. When we fast, our bodies enter a state of ketosis, where ketones are produced as an alternative fuel source for the brain. Ketones have been shown to provide a more efficient energy source, which can enhance mental clarity, focus, and overall brain function.

Moreover, fasting stimulates the production of a protein called brain-derived neurotrophic factor (BDNF), which plays a crucial role in promoting the growth and survival of neurons. BDNF is associated with improved memory, learning, and cognitive function. A study published in the Proceedings of the National Academy of Sciences (PNAS) demonstrated that fasting increased BDNF levels in the hippocampus, a region of the brain critical for memory formation.

Autophagy and Cellular Renewal: As we discussed earlier, fasting triggers a process called autophagy, which involves the breakdown and recycling of cellular components. This cellular "spring cleaning" allows the body to remove damaged proteins and organelles, promoting cellular renewal and overall health.

Autophagy has been linked to various health benefits, including a reduced risk of age-related diseases such as Alzheimer's and Parkinson's. Studies have shown that fasting can enhance autophagy and protect against the buildup of toxic protein aggregates in the brain. Additionally, autophagy plays a role in preventing cancer by eliminating damaged cells and inhibiting tumor growth.

Inflammation Reduction: Chronic inflammation is a common underlying factor in many diseases, including cardiovascular disease, diabetes, and autoimmune conditions. Fasting has been found to decrease inflammation markers in the body, potentially reducing the risk of developing these conditions.

By modulating the body's inflammatory response, fasting may contribute to better overall health and disease prevention.

Improved Longevity: Fasting has also been associated with increased lifespan and longevity. Studies conducted on various organisms, including yeast, worms, and flies, have shown that caloric restriction and intermittent fasting can extend lifespan and delay the onset of age-related diseases.

I While the direct evidence in humans is still limited, research suggests that fasting may activate longevity-related pathways and promote healthy aging. It is believed that the benefits of fasting, such as improved metabolic health, enhanced cellular repair, and reduced inflammation, contribute to the potential for increased lifespan.

Fasting has been found to have an impact on the production of growth hormone (GH) in the body. Growth hormone is a hormone secreted by the pituitary gland that plays a crucial role in growth, metabolism, and body composition. It promotes the growth of bone, muscle, and other tissues, as well as regulating metabolism and the breakdown of fats.

During periods of fasting, especially prolonged fasting, there is an increase in the secretion of growth hormone. This increase in growth hormone levels during fasting has been observed in several studies.

Intermittent Fasting (IF): This fasting method involves alternating between periods of fasting and eating. Common IF approaches include:
16/8 method: Fasting for 16 hours and restricting eating to an 8-hour window each day.
.

5:2 diet: Eating normally for five days of the week and restricting calorie intake to 500-600 calories on the remaining two non-consecutive days.

Extended Fasting: This refers to longer fasting periods, typically lasting 24 hours or more. It can be done occasionally or on a regular basis.

Time-Restricted Eating (TRE): This approach involves limiting daily food intake to a specific window of time, such as 8, 10, or 12 hours.

OMAD, which stands for "One Meal a Day," is a type of intermittent fasting where individuals consume all their daily calories in a single meal and fast for the remaining 22 hours of the day. It is a popular fasting approach that has gained attention for its simplicity and potential health benefits.

Chapter 9

How I Won The Battle

I want to share my personal journey of how I successfully won the battle against weight gain by combining the power of OMAD (One Meal a Day) and a low carb diet. It was a transformative experience that allowed me to regain control over my health, achieve my weight loss goals, and discover a newfound sense of well being. I hope that my story will inspire and motivate others who are on a similar journey towards a healthier lifestyle.

Like many others, I have struggled with weight gain throughout various phases of my life. Despite trying numerous diets and exercise programs, I found it challenging to achieve sustainable results. I felt trapped in a cycle of weight gain and loss, which took a toll on both my physical and emotional well-being. I knew I needed to find a different approach that would address the root causes of my weight gain and provide long-lasting results.

My breakthrough came when I discovered the concept of OMAD.

The idea of eating just one meal a day intrigued me, as it offered simplicity and flexibility.

I decided to give it a try, but I knew that to maximize the benefits, I needed to pair it with a nutrient rich and balanced diet. That's when I turned to a low carb approach.

A low carb diet focuses on reducing the intake of carbohydrates, particularly refined sugars and grains, while emphasizing whole foods rich in protein, healthy fats, and fiber. By minimizing carbohydrates, the body is encouraged to rely on stored fat for energy, leading to weight loss and improved metabolic health.

So combining OMAD with a low carb diet was a game changer for me. Not only did it simplify my eating routine, but it also allowed me to experience steady and sustainable weight loss. Here are some key aspects of my experience.

Black coffee is virtually calorie free, containing only a negligible number of calories per cup. During fasting, it's essential to avoid consuming any significant calories to maintain the fasting state. Choosing black coffee helps you stay hydrated and satisfied without breaking your fast.

Coffee, especially black coffee, contains caffeine, which is a natural appetite suppressant.

So I would have a black coffee at breakfast time and also at lunchtime to suppress my appetite,you can use green tea also but I prefer black coffee, very important no sugar no milk. Because black coffee can help reduce feelings of hunger and cravings, it can help to stick to your fasting schedule without feeling deprived or distracted by food.

The caffeine in black coffee provides a natural energy boost, which can help during fasting, especially if you experience temporary periods of low energy levels. This boost can help you stay focused and alert throughout your fasting window.

By keeping busy I use this strategy to support my fasting in various ways. Fasting can be challenging, especially during the initial stages, as your body adjusts to a new eating schedule. By staying busy, you can make fasting more manageable. Here are some ways in which I keeping busy can help with fasting.

One of the main challenges I've found is dealing with food cravings and thoughts of eating. When you keep yourself occupied with tasks, hobbies, work, or social activities, you have less time to dwell on food, making it easier to stick to your fast.

Staying busy can help you with mental focus and clarity during fasting. Engaging in activities that require concentration can shift your attention away from hunger or food-related thoughts, helping you stay on track with your fasting goals.

Remember that hunger comes in waves your body knows what time it wants to eat so you'll get hunger spikes generally throughout the day at breakfast time lunchtime and dinner time.

Fasting can sometimes affect mood, leading to irritability or low energy. Staying busy can help improve your mood and prevent feelings of boredom or frustration. So don't fall into the trap of feeling hangry. Now if you do not know what the the word hangry means I'll explain.

Hangry is a colloquial term that combines the words "hungry" and "angry" to describe a state of intense irritability or anger that is caused by hunger. When a person becomes hangry, they experience a shift in mood and behavior due to the physical sensations of hunger.

Chapter 10

The 12-week program

So you've got this far in the book now it's time for me to help you with program of devised to help you with this weight loss journey I understand that the program is not an easy journey but if you give me 12 weeks of your time you will reap the benefits. Now that we are embarking on it's not an easy path and you will feel like giving up and going back to your old eating habits but if you can stick to the program for the 12 weeks by the end of this period you will have a better understanding of your body and how you can continue with a healthy lifestyle with good weight management and longevity.

So this is not a diet I will not ask you to count calories or restrict calories Because I believe that this strategy doesn't work in the long term, yes you may get some short-term gains from calorie restrictions but you're not getting to the root of the problem, which is how we think about food. A strict calorie control diet may have some successes for a month or two, but then you slip back into your old habits and the weight will go back on, and you yo-yo same as always. That is why I do not believe in calorie control diets, and I think they do more harm than good.

I truly believe in a low calorie diet, you see all people are different, some people have a high tolerance for Carbohydrates. When I say some people I mean thin people, other people like us have a low tolerance for Carbohydrates. I only have to walk past a cake shop and I'll put on 5 kilos. So the remedy is low or minimal carbs, this program is not a calorie control diet, this is a program to help you with managing your carb intake. Once a week your weigh yourself either on a Saturday or a Sunday. Always try to make your weighing the same day and time to get consistency.

Week 1 and 2

Two Meals a Day (Lunch and Dinner)

During the first two weeks, you'll be gradually transitioning to a one meal a day approach or OMAD. Instead of starting with breakfast you have a black coffee or 2, you'll begin your eating window at lunchtime. This way, you can extend your overnight fasting period and give your body more time to burn stored fat for energy.

Finish dinner by around 8:00 PM. Aim for at least a 16 hour fasting window until your first meal at lunchtime the next day (around 12:00 PM).

Lunch

For your first meal, focus on protein-rich and nutrient-dense options to provide sustained energy.

Grilled chicken or turkey salad with mixed greens, cherry tomatoes, cucumbers, avocado, and olive oil dressing.

Baked salmon with roasted broccoli and cauliflower drizzled with lemon butter sauce.

Vegetarian option: Quinoa and chickpea salad with feta cheese, roasted red peppers, and a lemon-herb vinaigrette.

Dinner

For dinner, maintain a balanced meal with a focus on protein and healthy fats. Some ideas include:

Grilled steak with eggs a side of sautéed spinach and mushrooms in garlic butter.

Zucchini noodles (zoodles) with a creamy pesto sauce and grilled shrimp.

Stuffed bell peppers with ground turkey, cauliflower rice, and melted cheese on top.

Beverages

Stay hydrated throughout the day with water, herbal teas, and black coffee without added sugar or cream. Avoid sugary beverages, diet drinks and all fruit juice.

Remember, the key to success during the first two weeks is to stick to your chosen eating window and make mindful, nutritious food choices. Gradually reducing the eating window will help your body adjust to the new eating pattern, making the transition smoother.

Keep in mind that while low-carb meals can be beneficial for appetite control during fasting, it's essential to maintain a balanced diet that includes a variety of nutrient-dense foods. If you have any underlying health conditions or dietary restrictions, consult with a healthcare professional or registered dietitian before starting any new eating plan.

Week 3-4

Transition to One Meal a Day (OMAD)

In Weeks 3 and 4, we will take the next step in our fasting journey and shift to the One Meal a Day (OMAD) approach, making dinner the main meal of the day. OMAD with dinner allows you to enjoy a satisfying and fulfilling meal at the end of the day, making it easier to stick to the fasting schedule and maximize the benefits of intermittent fasting.

Start lunch at 2 PM and start diner at 6 PM.

In these two weeks is important to reduce the size of the lunchtime meal Because it's now we are on track to Omed.

Since dinner will be your main and only meal, it's crucial to make it nourishing and balanced, providing all the nutrients your body needs. Your dinner should include.

A generous portion of protein: Choose from options like grilled salmon, lean steak, chicken breast, or plant based proteins like tofu or tempeh.

Healthy fats: Incorporate sources like olive oil, avocado, nuts, or seeds for added flavor and satiety.

Non-starchy vegetables: Load up on nutrient-rich vegetables like spinach, Brussels sprouts, zucchini, or asparagus.

Low-carb side dishes: Consider cauliflower rice, spaghetti squash, or roasted sweet potatoes in moderation.

A refreshing salad: Complement your dinner with a colorful salad drizzled with a light vinaigrette.

Drink water or herbal tea during the meal to aid digestion and hydration.

Week 5-8

One Meal a Day (OMAD)

Transition to one meal a day, where you consume all your daily calories within a 1-2 hour eating window. Ensure that your single meal is nutritionally balanced and contains all essential nutrients.
Listen to your body's hunger cues and stop eating when you feel satisfied.

Week 9-10

Experiment with varying your eating window between 1-2 hours to keep your metabolism adaptable. Continue focusing on nutrient-dense whole foods to meet your nutritional needs.

Weeks 11-12

Introducing a Well-Deserved Cheat Day

Congratulations on reaching Weeks 11 and 12 of your fasting and low-carb journey! By now, you've mastered the art of intermittent fasting and embraced a healthy low-carb lifestyle. As we approach the end of the program, we will introduce a well-deserved cheat day to reward your efforts and help you maintain a positive relationship with food.

Cheat Day

Choose either a Saturday or a Sunday as your designated cheat day, depending on what day you typically weigh in or what works best for your schedule.

On your cheat day, you can enjoy some of your favorite treats and foods that you've been avoiding during the week. Indulge in moderation, savoring each bite mindfully.
Remember, the cheat day is not a day to binge or overeat; it's an opportunity to enjoy the foods you love without guilt. Listen to your body's signals and stop when you feel satisfied.

While you can have your favorite foods, remember to practice moderation. Enjoy a reasonable portion of each treat to prevent feeling overly stuffed or uncomfortable.
Balance your cheat day with healthy choices during your fasting period and other meals throughout the week.

Be mindful of how your body responds to different foods on your cheat day. Pay attention to how you feel, both physically and emotionally.
Notice any changes in your energy levels, mood, or cravings after indulging in certain foods. This awareness can help you make more informed choices in the future.

Throughout Weeks 11 and 12, continue your fasting and low-carb routine on non-cheat days. Stick to your regular fasting window and enjoy nutritious, low-carb meals.

Reflect on your progress and the positive changes you've experienced over the past weeks. Celebrate your achievements and be proud of the hard work you've put into your health and well-being.

At the end of Week 12, conduct a final weigh-in and assess your overall progress. Celebrate your successes, whether they be in terms of weight loss, improved energy, better sleep, or enhanced well-being.
Take some time to reflect on your journey and the lessons you've learned. Acknowledge the positive changes you've made to support your health and how you can continue to maintain these habits going forward.

As you move forward, feel free to continue incorporating a cheat day or adjust your approach based on what works best for you and your body. Trust yourself, be kind to yourself, and know that you have the power to maintain the healthy habits you've cultivated throughout this 12-week program. Congratulations on your achievements, and here's to a happier, healthier, and more balanced you!

Chapter 11

People That Have Had A Major influence Over Me

The first person I'd like to discuss is Dr Michael Mosley. Dr Michael Mosley is a name that has become synonymous with groundbreaking research, innovative health concepts, and transformative lifestyle changes. As a British medical doctor, journalist, and television presenter, Dr. Mosley has played a significant role in bringing cutting-edge medical knowledge to the masses, inspiring countless individuals on their journey to improve their health and well-being.

One of the most influential works of Dr. Mosley is his book "The Fast Diet," co-authored with Mimi Spencer. Published in 2013, this book introduced the concept of intermittent fasting, popularly known as the 5:2 diet. The premise of the 5:2 diet is to eat normally for five days a week and restrict calorie intake to 500-600 calories on the remaining two days. This approach captivated the world and sparked a widespread interest in the potential benefits of intermittent fasting for weight loss and overall health.

In "The Fast Diet," Dr. Mosley delves into the science behind intermittent fasting and explains how it can trigger beneficial changes in the body. He shares his own personal experience with fasting and how it transformed his own health, leading to weight loss, improved blood sugar levels, and increased energy. Dr. Mosley's storytelling style makes complex medical concepts accessible, engaging, and relatable to readers from all walks of life.

Following the success of "The Fast Diet," Dr. Mosley continued to explore the realms of health and nutrition, authoring several other influential books that have inspired millions worldwide.

Dr. Mosley's relentless pursuit of knowledge has not been confined to the pages of his books; he has also shared his wisdom through television documentaries and programs. "Eat, Fast & Live Longer," a Horizon documentary in which he explored the effects of fasting on longevity, was a landmark moment in his career. The documentary showcased his dedication to bridging the gap between scientific research and public understanding.

Dr. Mosley's work on intermittent fasting and gut health struck a chord with me, and I decided to incorporate these principles into my daily life. The 5:2 diet became a sustainable and effective way for me to manage my weight, and I noticed positive changes in my overall well-being. Embracing the principles of the Clever Guts Diet also allowed me to prioritize the health of my gut, leading to increased energy levels and improved digestion.

Beyond the scientific aspect of his work, Dr. Mosley's empathetic and down-to-earth approach touched my heart. He acknowledges that adopting new habits and making lifestyle changes can be challenging, and he gently encourages his audience to take small steps towards positive transformations. His openness about his own struggles and triumphs adds a human touch to his work, making readers and viewers feel like they have a trusted friend guiding them on their journey to better health.

His books and documentaries have influenced me deeply, guiding me on a path to weight loss and improved health. Through his work, I have discovered the immense power of knowledge and the potential for positive change that lies within us all.

The Diabetes Code" is another groundbreaking book by Dr. Fung that focuses on understanding and managing type 2 diabetes. Dr. Fung emphasizes the role of insulin in diabetes and proposes a transformative strategy to reverse the condition. Through therapeutic fasting and low-carb nutrition, he demonstrates how individuals with type 2 diabetes can regain control of their blood sugar levels and potentially eliminate the need for medication.

What sets Dr. Fung's work apart is his commitment to evidence-based research. He brings a wealth of scientific knowledge and clinical experience to his writing, making complex medical concepts accessible to the general public. As a result, his books resonate with readers from all walks of life, empowering them with the knowledge and tools to take charge of their health.

Personally, Dr. Jason Fung has had a profound impact on my weight loss journey. His clear and compelling explanations helped me understand the underlying causes of weight gain and how to overcome them. His emphasis on insulin resistance and the benefits of fasting inspired me to incorporate intermittent fasting into my daily routine, leading to significant improvements in my weight, energy levels, and overall health.

Dr. Jason Fung is a renowned Canadian nephrologist who has made significant contributions to the fields of fasting, intermittent fasting, and low-carbohydrate diets. His groundbreaking work has revolutionized the way we approach weight loss, diabetes management, and overall health. Through his books, lectures, and clinical practice, Dr. Fung has inspired countless individuals, including myself, on a journey to lose weight and improve their well-being.

One of Dr. Fung's most influential books is "The Obesity Code," a comprehensive guide that challenges conventional beliefs about weight loss. In this book, Dr. Fung delves into the root causes of obesity, debunking myths surrounding calorie counting and highlighting the critical role of hormones, particularly insulin, in weight gain. He introduces the concept of "insulin resistance," explaining how excessive insulin levels can prevent the body from burning fat effectively and lead to weight gain.

Dr. Fung's approach to weight loss centers around the idea of fasting as a powerful tool to improve metabolic health. In "The Complete Guide to Fasting," he provides a detailed overview of different fasting methods.

Through learned to prioritize nutrient-dense, whole foods while reducing my carbohydrate intake. I discovered that by adopting a low-carb lifestyle and embracing fasting as part of my routine, I could achieve sustainable weight loss and experience numerous health benefits.

Dr. Jason Fung's groundbreaking work on fasting, low-carb nutrition, and metabolic health has been an inspiration to many, myself included. Through his books and teachings, he has empowered individuals to take control of their health, challenge conventional wisdom, and achieve sustainable weight loss and improved metabolic health. Dr. Fung's impact on the field of health and nutrition is profound, and his legacy will continue to shape the way we approach weight loss and overall well-being for years to come.

The last mention in this chapter is Professor Tim Specter I've already mentioned professor Specter but I'll just go over a few more points

Professor Tim Spector is a highly respected genetic epidemiologist and researcher, known for his pioneering work in the field of personalized nutrition and gut health.

His book "The Diet Myth: The Real Science Behind What We Eat" has been a game-changer in the world of nutrition, challenging conventional beliefs about dieting and shedding light on the importance of individualized approaches to weight loss and overall health. Through his work, Professor Spector has influenced countless individuals, including myself, on a transformative journey to lose weight and achieve optimal well-being.

In "The Diet Myth," Professor Spector explores the complex interplay between our genes, gut microbiome, and diet, debunking common dieting myths and offering evidence-based insights into what truly matters for sustainable weight loss. He emphasizes that one-size-fits-all diets rarely work and that each person's response to food is unique, shaped by their genetics and gut microbes.

Personally, Professor Tim Spector's work has been a guiding light in my weight loss journey. His evidence-based approach and emphasis on personalized nutrition resonated with me, prompting me to reassess my own eating habits and prioritize gut health. His research-backed insights dispelled the notion of a one-size-fits-all diet and instead encouraged me to embrace a more flexible and intuitive approach to eating.

Bonus Chapter

Low Carbohydrate Recipes

light lunches

Grilled Eggplant and Zucchini Salad

Ingredients

1 large eggplant, sliced into rounds
2 medium zucchinis, sliced into rounds
100g cherry tomatoes, halved
50g Kalamata olives, pitted
50g feta cheese, crumbled
2 tablespoons balsamic vinegar
2 tablespoons olive oil
Fresh basil leaves for garnish
Salt and pepper to taste

Cooking Method

Preheat the grill or grill pan over medium-high heat.
Drizzle olive oil over the eggplant and zucchini slices, then sprinkle salt and pepper.
Grill the eggplant and zucchini slices for a few minutes on each side until they have grill marks and are tender.
In a bowl, mix grilled eggplant and zucchinis with halved cherry tomatoes and pitted Kalamata olives.
Drizzle balsamic vinegar over the salad and toss to combine.
Top with crumbled feta cheese and garnish with fresh basil leaves before serving.

Grilled Turkey and Vegetable Skewers

Ingredients

200g turkey breast (cut into cubes)
100g bell peppers (cut into chunks)
100g zucchini (cut into rounds)
100g cherry tomatoes
1 tablespoon olive oil
1 teaspoon dried oregano
1 teaspoon paprika
Salt and pepper to taste

Cooking Method

Preheat the grill or barbecue to medium-high heat.
In a bowl, toss the turkey cubes, bell peppers, zucchini, and cherry tomatoes with olive oil, dried oregano, paprika, salt, and pepper.
Thread the turkey and vegetables onto skewers alternately.
Grill the skewers for about 10 minutes, turning occasionally, until the turkey is cooked through and the vegetables are tender.
Serve hot.

Grilled Chicken Salad

Ingredients:

200g boneless, skinless chicken breast
100g mixed salad greens (lettuce, spinach, arugula)
50g cherry tomatoes, halved
50g cucumber, sliced
30g red onion, thinly sliced
20g feta cheese, crumbled
2 tablespoons olive oil
1 tablespoon lemon juice
Salt and pepper to taste

Cooking Method

Preheat the grill or grill pan over medium-high heat.
Season the chicken breast with salt and pepper.
Grill the chicken breast for about 6-7 minutes on each side or until fully cooked.
Let the chicken rest for a few minutes before slicing it into strips.In a large bowl, combine the mixed salad greens, cherry tomatoes, cucumber, and red onion. Whisk together olive oil, lemon juice, salt, and pepper to create the dressing. Drizzle the dressing over the salad and toss to coat. Top the salad with grilled chicken strips and crumbled feta cheese.
Serve as a protein-packed and refreshing lunch option.

Stuffed Bell Peppers with Cauliflower Rice

Ingredients

4 large bell peppers (any color you prefer)
300g cauliflower rice (store-bought or homemade)
250g lean ground beef (or turkey)
1 small onion, finely chopped
2 cloves garlic, minced
1 cup diced tomatoes (canned or fresh)
1 tablespoon tomato paste
1 teaspoon ground cumin
1 teaspoon paprika
1/2 teaspoon chili powder (optional for heat)
Salt and pepper to taste
1 cup grated cheese (cheddar, mozzarella)

Cooking Method

Preheat the oven to 180°C (356°F). Cut the tops off the bell peppers and remove the seeds and membranes. If needed, trim the bottom slightly to create a flat surface so the peppers can stand upright. In a large pan, brown the ground beef (or turkey) over medium-high heat until fully cooked. Drain any excess fat if necessary. Add the chopped onion and minced garlic to the pan with the cooked meat. Sauté for a few minutes until the onions are translucent and fragrant.

Stir in the diced tomatoes, tomato paste, ground cumin, paprika, chili powder (if using), salt, and pepper. Cook for another 2-3 minutes to let the flavors meld. Add the cauliflower rice to the pan and mix it well with the meat and spice mixture. Cook for an additional 3-4 minutes until the cauliflower rice is heated through. Stuff the bell peppers with the cauliflower rice and meat mixture, pressing it down gently to fill the peppers. Place the stuffed bell peppers in a baking dish. If there is any leftover cauliflower rice mixture, you can add it around the bell peppers. Sprinkle grated cheese over the top of each stuffed pepper. Cover the baking dish with aluminum foil and bake in the preheated oven for about 25-30 minutes, or until the peppers are tender and the cheese is melted and bubbly. Remove the foil and bake for an additional 5-7 minutes to lightly brown the cheese. Serve the stuffed bell peppers with cauliflower rice immediately.

To Make Cauliflower Rice, Follow These Steps

Rinse a cauliflower head and pat it dry with a paper towel.

Remove the leaves and stem from the cauliflower, leaving only the florets.

Cut the cauliflower into smaller pieces to fit into a food processor or use a box grater.

If using a food processor, place the cauliflower pieces in the processor bowl and pulse a few times until the cauliflower resembles rice grains. Be careful not to overprocess, as it may turn mushy.

If using a box grater, rub the cauliflower pieces against the large holes of the grater to create rice-like bits.

Once the cauliflower is riced, it can be used in various dishes as a rice substitute, such as stir-fries, fried rice, stuffed vegetables, and more.

Tuna Avocado Boats

Ingredients

2 ripe avocados
200g canned tuna, drained
30g red bell pepper, diced
30g celery, diced
2 tablespoons mayonnaise
1 tablespoon lemon juice
Salt and pepper to taste
Fresh parsley for garnish

Preparation Method

Cut the avocados in half and remove the pit. Scoop out a bit of flesh from each half to create a larger cavity for the tuna filling.
In a bowl, combine the canned tuna, diced red bell pepper, diced celery, mayonnaise, lemon juice, salt, and pepper.
Mix everything together until well combined.
Spoon the tuna mixture into the hollowed-out avocados.
Garnish with fresh parsley before serving.

Shrimp and Avocado Ceviche

Ingredients

150g cooked shrimp (peeled and deveined)
2 ripe avocados (diced)
1 small red onion (finely chopped)
1 small tomato (diced)
1 chili pepper (finely chopped, optional for heat)
Juice of 2 limes
2 tablespoons fresh cilantro (chopped)
Salt and pepper to taste

Cooking Method

In a bowl, combine the cooked shrimp, diced avocados, finely chopped red onion, diced tomato, and chopped chili pepper (if using).
Squeeze the lime juice over the mixture and toss gently to combine.
Season with salt and pepper to taste.
Sprinkle chopped cilantro over the top before serving.

Egg and Spinach Omelette

Ingredients

4 eggs
50g fresh spinach leaves
30g feta cheese (crumbled)
10g butter
Salt and pepper to taste

Cooking Method

In a bowl, beat the eggs until well combined. Season with salt and pepper.
In a non-stick frying pan, melt the butter over medium heat. Add the fresh spinach leaves to the pan and sauté until wilted. Pour the beaten eggs over the spinach. Sprinkle the crumbled feta cheese over one half of the omelette. Once the eggs are set, fold the omelette in half to cover the filling.
Slide the omelette onto a plate and serve hot.

Grilled Chicken with Pesto Sauce

Ingredients

2 chicken breasts (about 150g each)
50g fresh basil leaves
30g grated Parmesan cheese
30g pine nuts
2 cloves garlic
3 tablespoons olive oil
Salt and pepper to taste

Cooking Method

Preheat the grill or barbecue to medium-high heat.
Season the chicken breasts with salt and pepper.
In a blender or food processor, combine the fresh basil leaves, grated Parmesan cheese, pine nuts, garlic, and olive oil to make the pesto sauce.
Grill the chicken breasts for about 6-8 minutes on each side until fully cooked.
Serve the grilled chicken with a drizzle of pesto sauce on top.

Main Meal Recipes

Baked Lemon Herb Salmon

Ingredients

2 salmon fillets (about 150g each)
1 lemon (sliced)
2 tablespoons olive oil
1 tablespoon fresh dill (chopped)
1 tablespoon fresh parsley (chopped)
Salt and pepper to taste

Cooking Method

Preheat the oven to 200°C (392°F).
Place the salmon fillets on a baking sheet lined with parchment paper.
Drizzle olive oil over the salmon and season with salt and pepper.
Arrange lemon slices on top of the salmon.
Sprinkle chopped dill and parsley over the salmon.
Bake in the preheated oven for about 15-20 minutes or until the salmon is cooked through and flakes easily with a fork.
Serve hot.

Thai Basil Chicken (Pad Krapow Gai)

Ingredients

200g chicken breast (minced or thinly sliced)
1 tablespoon vegetable oil
2 cloves garlic (minced)
1 red chili (sliced, seeds removed for less heat)
1 tablespoon fish sauce
1 tablespoon oyster sauce
1 tablespoon soy sauce
1 teaspoon sugar substitute (such as erythritol or stevia)
1 cup fresh Thai basil leaves

Cooking Method

Heat the vegetable oil in a wok or large pan over medium high heat. Add the minced chicken and stir-fry until cooked and slightly browned. Add the minced garlic and sliced red chili to the pan and continue to stir fry for another minute until fragrant. In a small bowl, mix together the fish sauce, oyster sauce, soy sauce, and sugar substitute to make the sauce. Pour the sauce over the chicken and stir to combine. Add the fresh Thai basil leaves to the pan and toss everything together until the basil is wilted. Serve hot with cauliflower rice or zucchini noodles.

Lemon Herb Grilled Chicken Skewers

Ingredients:

2 chicken breasts (about 150g each)
1 lemon (juice and zest)
2 tablespoons olive oil
1 tablespoon fresh thyme (chopped)
1 tablespoon fresh rosemary (chopped)
Salt and pepper to taste

Cooking Method

Cut the chicken breasts into cubes and place them in a bowl. In a separate bowl, mix together the lemon juice, lemon zest, olive oil, chopped thyme, chopped rosemary, salt, and pepper to make the marinade. Pour the marinade over the chicken cubes and toss to coat evenly. Let it marinate in the refrigerator for at least 30 minutes. Preheat the grill or barbecue to medium-high heat. Thread the marinated chicken cubes onto skewers. Grill the chicken skewers for about 8-10 minutes, turning occasionally, until fully cooked and slightly charred.
Serve hot.

Thai Green Papaya Salad (Som Tum)

Ingredients

200g green papaya (shredded)
2 cloves garlic (minced)
1-2 Thai red chilies (sliced, seeds removed for less heat)
2 tablespoons fish sauce
1 tablespoon lime juice
1 teaspoon sugar substitute (such as erythritol or stevia)
50g cherry tomatoes (halved)
20g roasted peanuts (crushed)
Fresh cilantro for garnish

Cooking Method

In a mortar and pestle, pound the minced garlic and sliced Thai red chilies to release their flavors. Add the shredded green papaya to the mortar and gently pound to bruise the papaya and allow it to absorb the flavors. In a small bowl, mix together the fish sauce, lime juice, and sugar substitute to make the dressing. Pour the dressing over the papaya and toss to combine. Add the halved cherry tomatoes to the salad and toss gently. Transfer the salad to a serving plate and garnish with crushed roasted peanuts and fresh cilantro.

Thai Grilled Beef Salad (Yam Nuea Yang)

Ingredients

200g beef steak (sirloin or ribeye)
1 tablespoon vegetable oil
1 cucumber (sliced)
1 small red onion (thinly sliced)
1 tomato (cut into wedges)
2 spring onions (sliced)
1 tablespoon fresh cilantro (chopped)
1 tablespoon fresh mint leaves (chopped)
Juice of 1 lime
2 tablespoons fish sauce
1 teaspoon sugar substitute 1 red chili

Cooking Method

Rub the beef steak with vegetable oil and season with salt and pepper. Grill the beef over high heat for about 3-4 minutes on each side or until desired doneness. Let the beef rest for a few minutes before slicing thinly. In a large bowl, combine the sliced beef, cucumber, red onion, tomato, spring onions, cilantro, and mint leaves. In a small bowl, whisk together the lime juice, fish sauce, and sugar substitute to make the dressing. Pour the dressing over the salad and toss to combine. Garnish with sliced red chili before serving.

Tandoori Chicken

Ingredients

500g chicken drumsticks or thighs
150g plain Greek yogurt
2 tablespoons lemon juice
2 tablespoons tandoori masala spice blend
1 tablespoon ginger-garlic paste
1 tablespoon vegetable oil
Salt to taste
Fresh coriander leaves for garnish
Lemon wedges for serving

Cooking Method

In a bowl, mix together Greek yogurt, lemon juice, tandoori masala spice blend, ginger-garlic paste, vegetable oil, and salt to make the marinade.
Add the chicken drumsticks or thighs to the marinade and coat them thoroughly. Let the chicken marinate in the refrigerator for at least 2 hours, or preferably overnight. Preheat the oven to 200°C (392°F).
Place the marinated chicken on a baking tray lined with parchment paper.Bake the chicken in the preheated oven for about 25-30 minutes or until fully cooked and charred on the edges.Garnish with fresh coriander leaves and serve with lemon wedges.

BBQ Pork Skewers

Ingredients

300g pork tenderloin (cut into cubes)
2 tablespoons BBQ sauce (look for a low-carb, sugar-free option)
1 tablespoon olive oil
1 teaspoon paprika
1/2 teaspoon garlic powder
Salt and pepper to taste

Cooking Method

In a bowl, mix together the BBQ sauce, olive oil, paprika, garlic powder, salt, and pepper.
Add the pork cubes to the bowl and toss them to coat with the marinade. Let the pork marinate in the refrigerator for at least 30 minutes.
Preheat the grill to medium-high heat.
Thread the marinated pork cubes onto skewers.
Grill the pork skewers for about 4-5 minutes on each side, or until the pork is fully cooked and has grill marks.
Serve hot.

Lamb Rogan Josh

Ingredients

500g boneless lamb shoulder
150g plain Greek yogurt
100ml heavy cream
1 tablespoon ginger-garlic paste
1 tablespoon garam masala
1 tablespoon ground coriander
1 tablespoon ground cumin
1 teaspoon chili powder
1 tablespoon vegetable oil
Salt to taste

Cooking Method

n a bowl, mix together Greek yogurt, ginger-garlic paste, garam masala, ground coriander, ground cumin, chili powder, heavy cream, and salt to make the marinade. Add the lamb pieces to the marinade and coat them thoroughly. Let the lamb marinate in the refrigerator for at least 2 hours, or preferably overnight. In a pan, heat vegetable oil over medium heat. Add the marinated lamb pieces to the pan and cook until the lamb is fully cooked and tender. Stir in heavy cream and simmer for an additional 2 minutes. Garnish with fresh coriander leaves before serving. Serve hot.

Butter Chicken (Murgh Makhani)

Ingredients

500g boneless, skinless chicken thighs
150g tomato puree
100g unsalted butter
100ml heavy cream
1 tablespoon ginger-garlic paste
1 tablespoon garam masala
1 tablespoon ground cumin
1 tablespoon ground coriander
1 teaspoon chili powder
Salt to taste

Cooking Method

In a pan, melt half of the unsalted butter over medium heat.Add ginger-garlic paste and sauté for a minute until fragrant. Stir in the tomato puree, ground cumin, ground coriander, garam masala, chili powder, and salt. Cook the sauce for about 5 minutes, until the oil starts to separate from the sauce. Add the chicken pieces to the sauce and cook until the chicken is fully cooked and tender. Stir in the remaining unsalted butter and heavy cream. Simmer the curry for an additional 5 minutes.Garnish with fresh coriander leaves before serving.Serve hot.